Low

CW01468572

Low Carb: Fat Burning, Delicious Low Carb Recipes for Breakfast, Lunch & Dinner

*(*Nutritious Meals for Daily Living*)*

Marco Barrett

Published by Jason Thawne
Publishing House

© Marco Barrett

Low Carb: Fat Burning, Delicious Low Carb
Recipes for Breakfast, Lunch & Dinner
(Nutritious Meals for Daily Living)

ISBN 978-1-989749-25-8

This document is geared towards providing exact and reliable information in regards to the topic and issue covered. The publication is sold with the idea that the publisher isn't required to render accounting, officially permitted, or otherwise, qualified services. If advice is necessary, legal or even professional, a practiced individual in the profession should be ordered.

- From a Declaration of Principles which was accepted and approved equally by a Committee of the American Bar Association and a Committee of Publishers and Associations.

The information provided herein is stated to be truthful and consistent, in that any liability, in terms of inattention or otherwise, by any usage or abuse of any policies, processes, or directions contained within is the solitary and also utter responsibility of the recipient reader. Under no circumstances will any legal responsibility or blame be held against the publisher for any reparation, damages, or monetary loss due to the information herein, either directly or indirectly.

Respective authors own all copyrights not held by the publisher.

The information herein is offered for just informational purposes solely, and is universal as so. The presentation of the information is without contract or any type of guarantee assurance.

The trademarks that are used are without any consent, and also the publication of the trademark is without permission or backing by the trademark owner. All trademarks and brands within this book are for clarifying purposes only and are the owned by the owners themselves, not affiliated with this document.

TABLE OF CONTENTS

Part 1

Introduction

We may not like the word "fat" but surprisingly, it is one of the most essential macronutrients our body requires in order to survive. The trick is to consume a small amount of healthy fats within your daily meals but more than anything it's about the 'type' of fats you consume. The type of fats you need to avoid are saturated fats as too much saturated fat can contribute to high cholesterol which increases the risk of heart disease, stroke and cardiovascular disease. Its recommended that you take in no more than 30g saturated fat per day. Saturated fats are found predominantly in animal meats, butter, lard, cream, meat (sausages, bacon), chocolate and biscuits. When you look at how much of each of the macronutrients you should consume within your diet per meal, the eat well

1

plate recommends to consume 50% Carbohydrates, 35% Protein and 15% Fat. This makes sense as over half of your plate should be made up of complex carbohydrates which are our main source of energy, over a quarter of the plate should be made up of protein which serves many roles including helping to make you feel full and a small amount of unsaturated fat. Fats are essential to us and we need them for several reasons. A small amount of unsaturated fats is vital for your health as they help your body to absorb fat soluble vitamins such as vitamin A, D and E and they can only be absorbed with the help of other fats. We also use fat as an energy source, but it's important to note that your body will always look to use carbohydrates (glycogen) as its main energy source first and when the glycogen stores become depleted the body will start to utilize fat for energy. Most people are ruing the excess fat that's settled in certain parts of their body, making it difficult for them to fit into those fabulous clothes they had bought a few years back. On the other hand, some people are so lean that they get exhausted after just a few hours' work and need some flesh on their bones to look healthier and more attractive. So just as important as it is for some people to lose weight, it's as equally important for some people to gain weight. One of the best ways to consume the necessary amount of fat is to eat right. If you are suffering from excess weight, have been hitting the gym and are reasonably active in your day-to-day life, but are still unable to shed those extra kilos, then you should focus on the quantity and types of foods that you're eating. Think of your body as a car, we use food as fuel and if we put the wrong types of food or fuel in our car it wouldn't respond well would it? Our body needs organic and essential nutrients to run efficiently, we need complex carbohydrates found in brown starchy foods full of fibre as

3

they digest slowly so that you can sustain high energy levels throughout the day. Not only that, when you eat foods rich in fibre it helps to give you that feeling of fullness and keeps the hunger pangs away, whereas if you're always eating simple white type of carbohydrates, they won't keep you full for long because they're broken down into sugars (glucose) very quickly and if you don't use the energy immediately it'll be stored as fat.

It's simple logic when you think about it, but our brains are pre-programmed to eat a certain way since birth and throughout our childhood. What our parents feed us becomes the norm and we carry the same eating habits into adulthood. It's important to note that, we don't just get fat by eating fat, we can get fat by over consumption of carbohydrates and protein. In most cases it's usually too much carbohydrates and of the simple sort. It's given the term 'simple' because they're easily broken down, digested and absorbed into the bloodstream quickly to use as energy. Everything we eat is broken down into glucose which is sugar to use as energy but depending on the type of carbohydrate determines how slow or fast the energy is released. Simple carbohydrates can be very healthy and beneficial for the body when eaten at the right time. As you know fibre is digested slowly which releases energy slowly so if you are quite sedentary and don't exercise your diet should consist predominantly of complex carbohydrates rich in fibre. Or, even if you are sedentary and you exercise, simple carbohydrates can serve an important purpose after exercise. Right after exercise our body and muscles are like magnets for a small amount of simple carbohydrates because they need to be refuelled with glycogen to repair, grow and to refuel, we also need a decent amount of protein which also helps the repair and growth process of the muscles. It's best to have about 0.5-1 cup of white pasta for example as a portion size right after exercise and again 1-2 hours later. If you were to consume complex carbohydrates after exercise your body wouldn't get the nutrients it requires right away to repair and refuel therefore it will look to breakdown muscle tissue for energy, so essentially your body would be in starvation mode, this can lead to severe fatigue.

This book contains a host of recipes, some simple and some fit for a family meal, which will help you to boost your metabolism and burn body fat faster. So you don't have to starve while you get that fit body; you just need to keep a close eye on what you eat and know how many calories you are consuming in that one meal. To help with this, I have broken down the nutrition value of each recipe so that you know exactly how many calories you're taking in and exactly how many of them are from protein, carbohydrates and fat.

White Bean, Herbed Hummus and Crudités

Serves: 1
Preparation Time: 5 minutes
Ingredients:
¼ cup white beans, rinsed and drained
- 1 tbsp. chives, chopped
- 1 tbsp. lemon juice
- 2 tbsp. Olive oil

Nutrition info:
Protein – 6.1g
Carbohydrates – 14.1g
Fat – 27.5g
Total kcals – 328.3 Kcals
Raw vegetables as per choice, such as ripe tomatoes, green and red peppers, carrots and broccoli florets
Method:

In a large bowl, mix the beans, chives, lemon juice and olive oil well together, mashed, to form a paste.

1. Serve the paste along with the raw vegetables. You can also have other fresh fruits and vegetables in combination with this dish, such as cucumbers, radish, etc. as per taste.

USP: This is extremely easy to prepare and a light dish with a lot of good fat and none of the bad ones.

Rice Salad, Middle Eastern Style

Serves: 4
Preparation Time: 15 minutes
Ingredients:
¾ cup chopped Vidalia or sweet onion

- 16 ounces of chickpeas (one can is equivalent of this measurement), rinsed and drained
- 800g cooked brown rice
- ½ cup chopped pitted dates
- ¼ cup fresh mint, finely chopped
- ¼ cup fresh parsley, finely chopped
- ½ tsp. Cumin powder
- ¼ tsp. Salt
- Some black pepper, to taste

Nutrition info:
Protein – 45.5g / 11.4 per serving
Carbohydrates – 358.8g / 89.7g per serving
Fat – 11.5g / 2.9g per serving
Total Kcals – 1720.7 Kcals / 430.2 Kcals
Method:

In a large non-stick pan or skillet, heat the oil over medium heat and add the chopped onion. Stir the onion over flame until it turns golden brown. Turn off the flame and add the chickpeas, slat and cumin to it. Stir them all together well and when done, remove from heat. Add the ground pepper once the skillet is off the stove.

1. Take a large bowl and add all the ingredients together with the seasoned fried onions. Mix them all well together and serve the dish at room temperature.

USP: A welcome change to bland dietary fare, this dish contains a hint of flavour with zero cholesterol and lots of proteins and healthy fat.

3)
Toast with Broccoli and Feta Omelette

Serves: 1

Preparation Time: 7 minutes

Ingredients:

1 cup chopped broccoli

- 2 large beaten eggs
- 2 tbsp. crumbled feta cheese
- ¼ tbsp. dried dill
- 2 rye wheat bread slices, toasted
- Cooking Spray

Nutrition info:

Protein – 34.6g

Carbohydrates – 57.7g

Fat – 21.7g

Total Kcals – 564.5 Kcals

Method:

Place a non-stick skillet or pan over medium flame. Coat the vessel with the cooking spray. Add the chopped broccoli and cook it for about 3 minutes, while you stir the pieces enough so they don't stick to the bottom of the pan.

1. Mix the beaten egg, cheese and dill in a separate bowl very well so the omelette turns out soft and fluffy. Add this mixture to the pan and let is cook for 3-4 minutes. Once one side is cooked, flip the omelettes so both sides are evenly cooked. Serve this omelette with the toasts.

USP: This is a nutritious breakfast that doesn't require too many fruits and vegetables yet provides enough energy to last a while.

4) Breakfast Egg Pizza

Serves: 1
Preparation Time: 10 minutes
Ingredients:
1 egg, large
- 5 egg whites
- 2 tsp Grated Parmesan cheese
- ¼ cup grated zucchini
- 1/3 cup pasta sauce (select the one with the least amount of sodium in it)
- 1 tbsp. coconut flour
- Pizza seasonings as per taste
- Cooking spray

Nutrition info:
Protein – 32.5g
Carbohydrates – 17.1g
Fat – 11.7g
Total Kcals – 303.7 Kcals
Method:
Take a large skillet. Coat it with cooking spray. In a separate bowl, mix all the eggs, zucchini, coconut flour and pizza seasoning to make a fine batter and pour it in the coated skillet. Place it on medium heat.

1. Cover the skillet and let the eggs cook until the edge of the egg pizza turns light golden brown and crisp.
2. Put the grated cheese and pasta sauce on it. Your egg pizza is ready to be served, hot.

USP: The dish can be topped with lean meats of your choice, if you want to make your breakfast a little more protein rich.

5) Bok Choy with Garlic Recipe

Serves: 1
Preparation Time: 25 minutes
Ingredients:
1 Bok Choy head (a type of Chinese cabbage)
- 1 tbsp. red pepper, minced.
- 1 heaping tbsp. minced garlic
- 2 tbsp. soy sauce
- 2 tbsp. red wine vinegar
- 2 tbsp. olive oil
- Salt and pepper as per your taste preferences

Nutrition info:
Protein – 16.6g
Carbohydrates – 21.8g
Fat – 28.7g
Total Kcals – 411.9 Kcals
Method:
Shred the Bok choy and keep the pieces aside. In a separate, large bowl, make a sauce of the rest of the ingredients and when all have been thoroughly mixed,

soak the shredded Bok choy and let it remain soaked for 2 minutes.

1. Place the marinated Bok choy pieces in a baking tray and spoon the remaining sauce over them. Bake in a microwave oven for about 20 minutes at 350 degrees Celsius and serve the dish hot.

USP: An Oriental dish with a lot of flavour and immunity-building properties.

6) Crock pot turkey meat balls with green peppers

Serves: 4

Preparation Time: 7 hours

Ingredients:

450g lean minced turkey

- 2 medium onions, chopped
- 2 eggs
- 2 chopped green peppers
- 2 tbsp. coconut flour
- 1 head of cauliflower
- 1 bottle chilli sauce
- 1 can jelled cranberry sauce
- ½ cup Worcestershire sauce
- Cajun seasoning, salt, pepper and a pinch of seasoned salt

Nutrition info:

Protein – 125.9g / 31.5g per serving

Carbohydrates – 182.3g / 45.6g per serving

Fat – 58.4g / 14.6g per serving

Total Kcals – 1758.4 Kcals / 439.6 Kcals per serving

Method:

Cut the cauliflowers and green peppers and keep aside. In a separate bowl, mix well the ground turkey, eggs, flour, onions, Worcestershire sauce, pepper and the other seasonings.

1. Once well mixed, start rolling them into meatballs. Place all the balls at the bottom of the crock pot and cover them with the chopped cauliflowers and green peppers.

2. Pour the cranberry sauce and then the chilli sauce on the mixture. Cover the mixture and let it cook on high flame in the crock pot for about 7 hours, depending on the kind of pot you have. Serve the dish hot.

USP: Although it takes a little longer to prepare this one, it's a wholesome and filling dish with lean meat, very little fat and hardly any calories. A perfect dish for festive seasons or for guests!

7) Avocado, Tomato and Tuna Salad

Serves: 2
Preparation Time: 10 minutes
Ingredients:
150g tuna steak
- 8 asparagus tips
- 2 large tomatoes
- 150g lima beans, pre-cooked, rinsed and drained
- 1 small avocado
- 1 medium onion, thinly sliced
- 2 tbsp. extra virgin olive oil
- 1 tbsp. lemon juice
- 1 tbsp. fresh oregano, chopped
- 1 tsp Sea salt
- Black pepper

Nutrition info:
Protein – 55.1g / 27.5g per serving
Carbohydrates – 68.4g / 34.2g per serving
Fat – 44.8g / 22.4g per serving
Total Kcals – 897.2 Kcals / 448.6 Kcals per serving
Method:

Coat the tuna steaks with some of the olive oil and grill or dry fry them for about 3minutes. The outsides should turn firm and light golden brown but the inside should remain soft and pink so be careful not to grill the steaks for too long or use too much oil.

1. At the same time, put the asparagus in a microwave oven or steam it lightly until it turns tender. Chop the tomatoes and plate them along with the asparagus, onions and beans. Also cut the buttery part of the avocado into chunks and add them to the plate.

2. Add together the remaining oil, lemon juice, oregano and any other seasoning you may want to add, after you have added the sliced tuna steaks to the salad. Drizzle any remaining oil and seasoning on top, if required.

USP: This is a no carb, light flavoursome salad that will satisfy both your taste buds and your tummy! This energy packed, tasty salad can be taken with you anywhere, so prep a couple and take them with you on your travels.

8) Lemon Thyme Roast Chicken

Serves: 1

Preparation Time: 2 hours 50 minutes

Ingredients:

450g roasting chicken

- 2 large lemons
- 6 peeled garlic cloves
- 1 tsp black pepper, preferably freshly ground
- 2 tsp dried thyme leaves (if you prefer to use fresh thyme, then have six 4" thyme sprigs)
- Extra thyme sprigs for garnishing

Nutrition info:

Protein – 51.2g

Carbohydrates – 2.1g

Fat – 28.1g

Total Kcals – 466.1 kcals

Method:

In the cavity of the chicken to be cooked, place half of the salt and pepper. Take the lemons and pierce each of them about 15 times and make sure they are pierced at least an inch each time. It is advisable to soften the lemons before they are pierced by rolling them on a countertop and gently pushing them with the heel of your hands. Place the pierced lemons inside the cavity along with 5 garlic cloves. The remaining garlic clove can be placed in the smaller cavity of the chicken. Truss the chicken well.

1. On the trussed (tied) chicken, sprinkle the remaining salt and pepper and put it in a roasting pan, breasts up. Roast the chicken for 2.5 hours so that the chicken is cooked thoroughly. To check if it has been well cooked, pierce a fork in the meat and its juices should run clear or you can insert a kitchen thermometer in the thickest portion of the chicken's thigh and it should have a reading of 180 degrees Fahrenheit. The chicken is to be roasted in a pre-heated oven of 350 degrees Fahrenheit.

2. Remove any chicken skin that may be there, the garlic and the lemons from

within the roasted chicken. Carve the meat, garnish and consume hot.

USP: It's meat but minimally cooked and flavoursome.

9) Chocolate and Banana Treat

Serves: 1

Preparation Time: 5 minutes

Ingredients:

2 tbsp. chocolate chips (select the chips based on the type of chocolate you prefer, such as milky, dark chocolate (healthier choice), etc.)

- 1 medium sized banana, cut into chunks.

Nutrition info:

Protein – 3.3g

Carbohydrates – 47g

Fat – 8.4g

Total Kcals – 276.8 Kcals

Preparation:

Heat the chocolate chips in a microwave oven or a non-stick vessel until they are completely liquefied. Be careful not to burn the melted chocolate.

1. Take pan off stove or out of the oven and dip the banana chunks in the liquefied chocolate. Enjoy it straight off the oven or freeze them for future use.

USP: One of the simplest ways to get instant energy and satisfy your cravings without any bad fats.

10) Banana and Almond Buttered Toast

Serves: 1

Preparation Time: 5 minutes

Ingredients:

1 large banana, chopped into chunks
- 2 tbsp almond butter
- 4 slices of rye bread, toasted

Nutrition info:

Protein – 19.1g

Carbohydrates – 121.9g

Fat – 23.4g

Total Kcals – 774.6 Kcals

Method:

Evenly spread the almond butter on two slices of rye bread. Place equal quantities of banana slices on both bread slices.

1. Place the other two empty slices on the covered slices and enjoy your toasted sandwiches.

USP: A healthy and fresh breakfast that jumpstarts your day on an energetic note.

11) Barbecued Turkey Burgers

Serves: 2 burger servings
Preparation Time: 10 minutes
Ingredients:
150g minced turkey
- 2 sesame seed buns, lightly toasted
- 4 sweet onion slices, lightly grilled
- 1 garlic clove, finely chopped
- ¼ tsp cumin, ground
- ½ tsp paprika
- ¼ cup barbecue sauce
- ¼ tsp ground black pepper
- A pinch of kosher salt

Nutrition info:
Protein – 40.5g / 20.2g per serving
Carbohydrates – 105.4g / 52.7g per serving
Fat – 18.1g / 9.1g per serving
Total Kcals – 746.5 Kcals / 373.2 Kcals
Method:
Take a medium sized bowl and mix together the ground turkey, garlic, cumin and paprika to form an even mixture.

Make 4 patties of the mixture, each about 4" thick, and season the patties with pepper and salt.

1. Grill the patties on medium-high flame for about 7-8 minutes until it is fully cooked. Place within burger buns and serve with other fillings and toppings, such as cucumber, tomatoes, onion and carrot slices.

USP: A filling meal that can be carried while you are leaving for office or want to grab a quick lunch at work.

12) Quinoa Meal

Serves: 1

Preparation Time: 5 minutes

Ingredients:

1 cup quinoa, cooked

- 1/3 cup of canned, low sodium, drained and rinsed black beans
- 1 small tomato, chopped
- 1 tsp olive oil
- 1 spring onion, finely sliced
- 1 tbsp. freshly squeezed lemon juice
- Salt and taste according to taste

Nutrition info:

Protein – 19.7g

Carbohydrates – 69.3g

Fat – 17.3g

Total Kcals – 511.7 Kcals

Method:

1. Take all the ingredients and mix them well in a large bowl. The mixture is a ready to be consumed!

USP: Easy to make and packs quite a punch when it comes to energy giving calories. So if you want to have a simple meal, then this is it for you.

13) Barley, Banana and Sunflower Seeds' Breakfast

Serves: 1
Preparation Time: 15 minutes
Ingredients:
1/3 cup of easy-to-cook pearl barley, uncooked
- 2/3 cup water
- 1 tbsp. sunflower seeds
- 1 medium sized banana, sliced
- 1 tsp honey

Nutrition info:
Protein – 18.4g
Carbohydrates – 137.4g
Fat – 16g
Total Kcals – 767.2 Kcals
Method:
Pour the water and barley in a microwave bowl and heat the mixture for about 6 minutes. Wait for the barley to cook fully.
1. Take out the bowl, add the rest of the ingredients on top of it or mix them all together (except the banana slices as they are to be added in the end) and

your nutritious bowl of cereal is ready for breakfast.

USP: Light breakfast that is also easy to digest, this recipe is more beneficial for people who have digestion issues as there is honey in it.

14) Sandwich of Curried Eggs

Serves: 1

Preparation Time: 5 minutes

Ingredients:

2 hardboiled eggs, cut into sizeable chunks

- 2 tbsp. of chopped red pepper
- 2 tbsp. of low-fat, plain Greek yoghurt
- ½ cup of fresh spinach, chopped
- 1 orange, peeled
- 2 rye bread slices, lightly toasted
- ¼ tsp curry powder
- Salt and pepper as per taste

Nutrition info:

Protein – 33.5g

Carbohydrates – 58.7g

Fat – 18.9g

Total Kcals – 538.9 Kcals

Method:

In a medium sized bowl, mix the chopped eggs, bell pepper, salt, pepper, curry powder and yoghurt to make the curried eggs.

1. On one toasted rye bread slice, make a layer using the spinach, add the curried eggs on top of it, cover with the other slice of bread and get your sandwich ready.
2. Serve this sandwich with the orange on the side.

USP: This is a good combination of flavours and iron-boosting spinach to make a perfect evening snack or breakfast.

15) Salmon Noodles

Serves: 2

Preparation Time: 15 minutes

Ingredients:

Soba buckwheat noodles (4 ounces) or whole wheat spaghetti

- 5 Ounces asparagus, cut into big pieces
- 1 salmon fillet, de-skinned, cut into 8 pieces
- ½ of small avocado, the pulp cut into medium sized chunks
- 4 ounces of cucumber (with skin preferably) cut into small pieces
- 1 tbsp. sesame oil (toasted)
- Zest and 3 tbsp. of lime juice (for which you will need 2-3 small limes)
- ¼ tsp kosher salt
- ¼ tsp fresh pepper
- Cooking spray

Nutrition info:

Protein – 49.6g / 24.8g per serving

Carbohydrates – 91.7g / 45.8g per serving

Fat – 33g / 16.5g per serving

Total Kcals – 862.2 Kcals / 431.1 Kcals per serving

Method:

In a large bowl, cook the noodles or spaghetti until soft (takes about 8 or 6 minutes, respectively). Remove the cooked strands of noodles or spaghetti with tongs and place in a strainer.

1. In the same water, add the cut asparagus and boil until they turn soft. This should take about 1.5 minutes. Rinse the cooked asparagus under cold water and keep aside.

2. Take a non-stick pan or skillet, coat with cooking spray and place on medium-high flames. Place the salmon pieces and cook for 2-3 minutes. Keep turning the sides so they don't get overcooked and both sides of all pieces are evenly cooked.

3. To make the vinaigrette, take the sesame oil, lime zest and juice, salt and pepper in a small bowl and whisk them well. To this mixture, add the strained noodles or spaghetti and cooked asparagus and mix well again.

4. To this new mixture, add the cucumber and avocado pieces and toss them lightly, like you would to make a salad. Before you plate, add the cooked salmon pieces to the mixture and serve at room temperature.

USP: A tangy dish with pieces of fish, this dish is perfect for a good afternoon lunch without feeling too heavy at the end of the meal.

16) Greek Yoghurt and Fruits Parfait

Serves: 2

Preparation Time: 5 minutes (5 hours of refrigeration)

Ingredients:

¾ cup of plain, non-fat Greek yoghurt

- 1 plum, chopped
- 1 nectarine, chopped
- 1 peach, chopped
- ¾ cup of puffed cereal rice
- 1 tbsp. ground flaxseeds
- 2 tbsp. of slithered almonds
- 1 tbsp. honey

Nutrition info:

Protein – 39.4g / 19.7g per serving

Carbohydrates – 213.7g / 106.8g per serving

Fat – 28.8g / 14.4g per serving

Preparation:

Take a tall glass or container (big enough to contain all the ingredients) and add half of the yoghurt, chopped fruits, cereal, nuts and syrup, layer by layer.

1. Repeat the same after one set of layers has been added in the container, to form another layer of the same ingredients. Make sure the honey, syrup or nectar is the top-most layer of the parfait.
2. Make the parfait crunchy by adding crushed puffed cereal rice on top of the syrup and refrigerate for 5 hours. Serve chilled.

USP: A colourful, nutritious and delicious treat, this can be your perfect accompaniment for other fruits or a stand-alone meal between lunch and dinner or just a casual lunch.

17) Chicken Chilaquiles and Black Beans

Serves: 6

Preparation Time: 30 minutes

Ingredients:

600g shredded chicken breasts (6 chicken fillets)

- 1 tin of black beans, rinsed and drained
- 1 can of salsa de chilli fresco
- 15 corn tortillas cut into 1" strips
- 4 ounces (about 1 cup) of shredded queso blanco
- 1 cup fat-free and less sodium chicken broth
- 1 cup onion, finely chopped
- 5 garlic cloves, finely cut or minced
- Cooking spray

Nutrition info:

Protein – 300g / 50g per serving

Carbohydrates – 449.4g / 74.9g per serving

Fat – 58.9g / 9.8g per serving

Total Kcals – 3527.7 Kcals / 587.9 Kcals

Method:

Keep the oven pre-heated at 450 degrees Fahrenheit. Place a large non-stick pan or skillet over medium-high flames and coat it with cooking spray. Add the onions and sauté lightly until they turn golden brown.

1. To this, add the cut garlic and sauté for another minute. Add the shredded chicken and mix well for about 30 seconds. Remove contents of the pan and place in a separate cooking vessel, such as a bowl.

2. To this mixture, add the chicken broth, salsa and beans and cook until the broth boils. Turn down the flame to simmer and let the mixture cook for 5 minutes. Stir occasionally.

3. In a baking tray (11"x7") coated with cooking spray, place half the tortilla strips and add the cooked chicken mixture, evenly spread, on them. Add another layer of tortillas on top of this, and then add a fourth layer of the remaining chicken mixture. Add the remaining chicken broth on top of all the layers. Sprinkle some grated

cheese, if desired, and place the baking tray in the pre-heated oven.

4. Let the mixture bake at 450 degrees Fahrenheit for about 10 minutes or till all ingredients fully cooked. The tortillas should be lightly browned and the cheese should have melted completely.

USP: A traditional Mexican breakfast dish, this is perfect to be had at any time of the day and is a good mixture of meat and vegetables.

18) South-Western Spicy Black Beans (with Chilli)

Serves: 4

Preparation Time: 25 minutes

Ingredients:

½ cup avocado pulp, cut into pieces

- Cilantro sprigs for dressing
- ¼ cup fresh coriander, finely chopped
- ¼ cup low fat sour cream
- 2 cans of black beans, rinsed and drained
- 2 tsp olive oil
- 1 large onion, finely chopped
- 1 cup jalapenos, chopped
- 1 large garlic clove, thinly sliced
- 2 tbsp. chilli powder
- 1 tsp ground cumin
- 450g tomatoes (for roasted soup)
- 450g red peppers (for roasted soup)

Nutrition info:

Protein – 68.4g / 17.1g per serving

Carbohydrates – 219g / 54.7g per serving

Fat – 47.3g / 11.8g per serving

Total Kcals – 1575.3 Kcals / 393.8 Kcals per serving

Method:

In a large non-sticky skillet or pan, heat the oil on medium-high flame and add the onion and jalapeno. Stir until they are softened (about 3 minutes).

1. Add the sliced garlic, cumin and chilli powder while stirring. Let the mixture cook for about a minute. Add the black beans and soup and let the mixture simmer for about 5 minutes. Stir occasionally. Add the chopped cilantro and keep stirring.

2. Let the mixture cook for another minute and then pour it into 4 bowls. To each bowl, add 1 heaped tbsp of sour cream, avocado pieces and cilantro sprigs as garnishing and serve hot.

USP: This spicy and tasty dish is perfect for a cold, wintry morning or night. Spice lovers will be glad to have a nutritious meal without adding too much fat.

19) Chicken Dumpling Soup

Serves : 4

Preparation Time : 50 minutes

Ingredients :

1 lb boneless chicken breasts (450g)
- 4 cups of water
- 3 tins of reduced sodium chicken broth
- 1 medium sized onion, finely chopped
- 4 carrots, chopped
- Fresh parsley, chopped
- ½ teaspoon salt
- ¼ teaspoon garlic seasoning
- ½ teaspoon pepper
- 1 cup all-purpose white wheat flour
- 3 eggs, only the white part
- 2 tablespoon water
- ½ cup cottage cheese

Nutrition info:

Protein – 187.2g / 46.8g per serving

Carbohydrates – 138.6g / 34.6g per serving

Fat – 39.4g / 9.8g per serving

Total Kcals – 1657.8 Kcals / 414.4 Kcals

Method:

Use a non-sticky skillet that is coated with cooking spray to cook chicken in this recipe. You must add water, vegetables and seasonings and bring the chicken pieces to a boil.

1. Keep stirring the contents of the vessel as you begin to reduce the heat and keep the dish uncovered for half an hour. This makes the vegetables tender and soft.

2. In a different container, add the whites of the eggs and beat them with cottage cheese until it is a smooth blend. When the mixture is frothy, you can add the flour as well and continue to blend it and create dumplings.

3. Boil the soup and drop in dumplings using a large handled spoon.

USP: For best taste, it is vital that you cover the dish for at least 15 minutes before it gets cold.

20) Zesty Diced Chicken

Serves: 4

Preparation Time: 20 minutes

Ingredients:

2 lbs boneless chicken pieces

- 2 tablespoons olive oil
- ½ cup orange juice
- 3 tablespoons soya sauce
- ¼ cup rice vinegar
- 3 tablespoons cornstarch
- 2 teaspoons ginger, finely ground
- ½ teaspoon white pepper
- 4 cloves of minced garlic
- ½ cup honey
- Salt to taste
- Orange zest and green onions, for garnishing

Nutrition info:

Protein – 216.8g / 54.2g per serving

Carbohydrates – 191.9g / 48g per serving

Fat – 41.7g / 10.4g per serving

Total Kcals – 2010.1 Kcals / 502.5 Kcals

Method:

Take a medium sized pan and heat oil over high heat. Add the boneless pieces of chicken and sauté it for about 5 minutes until the meat has a brownish sheen.

1. Add pepper and salt to taste.
2. Mix the garlic cloves, orange juice, honey, vinegar and soya sauce in a bowl. Add the corn starch and whisk it with pepper and finely ground ginger. Remember, if you prefer a sweeter version of the dish, then you can add some more honey to the mix.
3. Add the mixture of orange sauce onto the pan of chicken and stir until it has combined with the pieces of chicken. Allow it to simmer and come to a boil.
4. When the gravy is slightly thick, you can remove the chicken dish out of the flames and garnish it.
5. Serve this orange chicken with rice or eat it as a meal in itself.

21) Chicken Yoghurt Salad

Serves: 4

Preparation Time: 20 minutes

Ingredients:

1 pound shredded chicken pieces

- ½ cup apple, chopped
- ½ cup natural yoghurt
- Few cranberries
- ½ cup onion, diced
- Ten grapes, halved
- Few almonds for taste
- 1 tablespoon lime juice
- ½ teaspoon garlic powder
- Kosher salt to taste
- Sprinkle of black pepper, ground
- Bread, if preferred

Nutrition info:

Protein – 122.6g / 30.6g per serving

Carbohydrates – 110.8g / 27.7g per serving

Fat – 29.5g / 7.4g per serving

Total Kcals – 1199.1 Kcals / 299.7 Kcals per servings

Method:

For this salad, you have to first cook the chicken separately in a cooker or steam it in an appropriate vessel.

1. Add all the ingredients – the chicken, onion, apples, grapes, yoghurt, nuts, dried fruits and lime juice in a large bowl and whisk well.
2. Add salt to taste and garnish with pepper
3. You can have this salad as it is or combine it with ciabatta bread that is toasted lightly for a wholesome mean.

USP: This snack is a great substitute to energy bars that you consume before or after your workouts.

22) Chicken with Asparagus

Serves : 4

Preparation Time : 20 minutes

Ingredients:

1 lb boneless chicken breasts

- 2 tablespoons butter, low fat
- ¼ cup flour
- ½ teaspoon salt
- 1.5 cups asparagus, chopped
- 2 sliced lemons
- 2 tablespoons honey
- Parsley leaves for garnishing

Nutrition info:

Protein – 117.7g / 47.1g per serving

Carbohydrates – 106.9g / 26.7g per serving

Fat – 12.4g / 1.4g per serving

Total Kcals – 1009.3 Kcals / 252.3 Kcals per serving

Method:

Add the chicken boneless pieces into a bowl and mix it with salt and pepper.

1. Use some flour and toss all the pieces into this.
2. Keep a pan over medium heat and sauté the chicken pieces with the butter for five minutes until the meat is golden brown.
3. Transfer the chicken pieces into a plate.
4. Chop the asparagus and add it into the pan. Sauté until the vegetable becomes bright green and tender crisp.
5. Put the sliced lemon pieces on the pan and cook so that they caramelize lightly. You could add some butter while the lime slices are frying so that they do not stick to the pan.
6. You can now add the layer of asparagus onto the chicken and cover it with lemon slices.

USP: A recipe with short ingredient list, hence perfect for people who don't have time to lose themselves in a grocery shop.

23) Cauliflower Roast Snack

Serves: 4

Preparation Time: 20 minutes

Ingredients:

1 head of cauliflower

- 3 cloves of garlic, sliced
- ¼ lemon
- 3 tablespoons of parsley, chopped
- ½ cup tomatoes, chopped
- 2 tablespoons of extra virgin olive oil
- Salt to taste
- 2 teaspoons of black pepper, freshly ground

Nutrition info:

Protein – 18.8g / 4.7g per serving

Carbohydrates – 54.1g / 13.5g per serving

Fat – 28.2g / 7.1g per serving

Total Kcals – 545.4g / 136.3 Kcals per serving

Method:

Since this recipe consumes less oil, we shall bake the cauliflowers and hence preheat the oven to 220 degrees.

1. Add the tomatoes and cauliflowers with the olive oil and salt into the baking pan.
2. Allow the vegetables to bake until the cauliflower is brown and tender.
3. After about fifteen to twenty minutes, you can take the pan out and serve the cauliflowers with parsley and a few drops of lemon for a citric taste.

USP: Something unique happens when cauliflower is roasted – it starts to taste like popcorn. The flavour completely changes and the vegetable turns into something really delicious and healthy.

24) Easy Chicken Treats

Serves: 4

Preparation Time: 20 minutes

Ingredients:

400g of chicken breast pieces

- 3 cloves of garlic that are nicely minced
- 2 tablespoons of ginger, minced
- 20 ml soya sauce
- 30g sugar, granulated
- 400g broccoli
- Salt to taste
- Finely granulated pepper
- 2 tablespoons of corn starch
- 15ml dry sherry
- 3 tablespoon vegetable oil

Nutrition info:

Protein – 137.4g / 34.3g per serving

Carbohydrates – 112.2g / 28.1g per serving

Fat – 42g / 10.5g per serving

Total Kcals – 1376.4 Kcals / 344.1 Kcals per serving

Method:

Add chicken pieces, garlic cloves, minced ginger, and soy sauce in a bowl. Mix them well and add corn flour to act as a binding factor.

1. Allow the mixture to marinate at room temperature with water or chicken broth, both are perfectly all right.

2. Heat a non-stick vessel and add oil into the pan. Once it begins to simmer, you can add the stems of broccoli and stir fry it for a minute or two.

3. You can now add the remaining ingredients like the salt and pepper along with the garlic cloves. Continue stirring until the broccoli stems turn bright green.

4. Once you have transferred the contents of the pan into a container, add the marinated chicken over high heat. Use the remaining tablespoons of vegetable oil and stir fry chicken until it becomes golden brown. In a matter of five minutes, your dish will be ready to eat.

25) Soft Buttermilk Chicken

Serves: 4

Preparation Time: 20 minutes

Ingredients:

300g of boneless chicken, preferably breast pieces

- 1 egg
- ½ teaspoon Kosher salt
- 1 cup all purpose flour
- 2 cups buttermilk, reduced fat
- ½ teaspoon red pepper, ground
- 1 tablespoon canola oil
- 3 teaspoons black pepper, ground

Nutrition info:

Protein – 135.6g / 33.9g per serving

Carbohydrates – 286g / 71.5g per serving

Fat – 54.3g / 13.6g per serving

Total Kcals – 2175.1 Kcals / 543.8 Kcals per serving

Method:

Add buttermilk, egg and red pepper with the pieces of chicken to marinate it and keep it preserved in a locked plastic bag.

You can place it in the refrigerator for almost 5 hours. Remember to defrost it before use later.

1. When you are cooking the meal, you must preheat the oven to about 400 degrees.
2. Use the chicken that has been defrosted and place it in a tray.
3. Sprinkle the chicken with generous amounts of kosher salt and red pepper. Also add the flour and mix well.
4. Use a pan to sauté the chicken for about 5 minutes before baking it.
5. Once you have baked the dish, it can be eaten with rice or bread and a sauce.

USP: This recipe is flavourful and crispy; it is a great option for picnics

26) Chicken with Spinach Artichoke

Serves: 8

Preparation Time: 40 minutes

Ingredients:

8 pieces of chicken breasts

- 10 oz spinach
- ½ cup yoghurt
- ½ cup shredded mozzarella cheese
- 2 onions, chopped
- 12 oz artichoke hearts, drained
- 3 cloves of garlic, minced
- ½ cup Parmesan cheese
- ½ cup mayonnaise, light

Nutrition info:

Protein – 364.3g / 45.5g per serving

Carbohydrates – 84.5g / 10.6g per serving

Fat – 140.5g / 17.6g per serving

Total Kcals – 3059.2 Kcals / 382.4 Kcals per serving

Method:

This simple recipe involves a bit of baking and a great deal of mixing.

1. Start by preheating your oven to about 370 degree Fahrenheit.
2. You can coat the edges of your baking tray or pan with a layer of olive oil so that the food does not stick to the surface.
3. Place the breasts of the chicken and add salt and pepper.
4. Bake it for about 15 minutes and allow it to remain inside the oven.
5. Add the artichoke, cloves, cheese and mayonnaise together in a bowl and whisk it properly. The shallots can be added at the end.
6. Now add this freshly whisked mixture over the chicken pieces and continue the roasting process.
7. After 20 minutes, the recipe will be ready to be tasted.

USP: When you take a healthy dose that comprises of artichokes, chicken and spinach, you leave a plenty of room for a great dessert.

27) Lentil Soup

Serves: 4

Preparation Time: 30 minutes

Ingredients:

450g lentils

- 2 tablespoons olive oil
- 150g onions, finely chopped
- ½ teaspoon cumin, freshly ground
- ½ teaspoon coriander seeds, freshly ground
- 250g tomatoes, chopped
- Salt to taste
- 25g celery, chopped
- 25g carrots, chopped

Nutrition info:

Protein – 45.9g / 11.5g per serving

Carbohydrates – 133.1g / 33.3g per serving

Fat – 29.6g / 7.4g per serving

Total Kcals – 982.4 Kcals / 245.6 Kcals per serving

Method:

Boil six litres of water in a large vessel. Add the vegetables and olive oil.

1. The onions, carrots and celery must be chopped finely and the salt must be added for taste. This must be left simmering for about seven minutes at least.
2. Now add the tomatoes, lentil, broth, cumin and coriander. Stir well and continue to simmer.
3. Boil the mixture and reduce the heat as you cover and cook the soup until the lentils are tender. This continues up to half an hour until the broth has thickened in consistency. The soup is best enjoyed when served hot.

USP: In this recipe, lentils are coupled with the goodness of vegetables, which makes it a perfect family friendly dish. As it is simple, easy-to-throw and comforting, lentil soul makes a perfect weekday dinner!

28) Simple Salmon Bake

Serves : 4

Preparation Time : 25 minutes

Ingredients:

¼ cup of Mayonnaise, light

- 1 pound of salmon fish fillets (approx. 450g)
- Salt and pepper to taste
- 5 cloves of garlic
- Hint of ginger
- Hint of paprika

Nutrition info:

Protein – 104.7g / 26.2g per serving

Carbohydrates – 5g / 1.2g per serving

Fat – 88g / 22g per serving

Total Kcals – 1230.8 Kcals / 307.7 Kcals per serving

Method:

For baking a fish, we first need to preheat the oven to about 325 degree Fahrenheit.

1. Line your baking tray with a foil that is oiled so as to prevent the meat from sticking to the base of the vessel.

2. Place the fish and use salt, pepper, ginger and garlic to lend it a slight appeal
3. Ensure that the paprika is sprinkled over the fish before it bakes.
4. You can bake it in the hot oven for about twenty minutes without turning it.

USP: Although the recipe is so delicious, it pulls together in less than 30 minutes. This versatile fish is a simple and easy way to get more of heart healthy Omega 3 fatty acids in your body.

29) Green Eggs and Ham Breakfast

Serves: 1

Preparation Time: 15 minutes

Ingredients:

1 portabella mushroom cap (large)

- 2 egg whites
- 1 whole egg
- ¼ avocado, sliced thinly
- ½ tbsp olive oil, divided into two halves
- Salt, pepper, herbs and spices as per taste

Nutrition info:

Protein – 31g

Carbohydrates – 8.2g

Fat – 19g

Total Kcals – 327.8 Kcals

Method:

Keep the broiler pre-heated and keep a large baking tray lined.

1. Discard the mushroom stem and brush both sides of the cap with half of the olive oil. Sprinkle salt lightly on both sides and then place the mushroom in

the baking tray, the gill or the interior of the mushroom facing up while the rounded top is touching the tray. Broil both sides of the mushroom for 5 minutes each, so that the cap turns soft.

2. On a skillet placed on low-medium flame, add a mixture of the eggs and fry using remaining oil. The egg whites and the whole egg are to be whisked in a separate bowl. Scramble the egg mixture and when done, spread the scrambled eggs on the softened mushroom cap.

3. Serve dish hot, with the avocado slices, spices and herbs added on top of the dish.

USP: This healthy meal is full of protein but also provides energy with hardly any calories being added to your body.

30) Omelette, Italian style

Serves: 4

Preparation time: 20 minutes

Ingredients:

½ avocado, pulp thinly sliced

- 1 can black beans, rinsed and dried
- 4 whole eggs
- 4 egg whites
- Juice extracted from one whole lime
- 4 tbsp bottled salsa
- A hint of hot sauce
- Salt and pepper as per taste
- Cooking Spray

Nutrition info:

Protein – 90.7g / 22.7g per serving

Carbohydrates – 86.6g / 21.7g per serving

Fat – 39.4g / 9.8g per serving

Total Kcals – 1063.8 Kcals / 266 Kcals per serving

Method:

In a food processed, blend well the lime juice, black beans and hot sauce.

1. Place a non-stick pan or skillet over medium high flame and coat with cooking spray. In a separate bowl, mix the contents of one whole egg with one egg white, a part of the salt and pepper and whisk well. Fry this mixture on the skillet or pan.

2. When the omelette is about to be cooked, add one fourth portion of the blended black beans sauce and fold the cooked side of the eggs on it. Flip the omelette so the other side also gets cooked, with the black beans' sauce inside it.

3. Top this omelette, when cooked, with salsa, avocado and any other seasoning of your choice and serve hot. Repeat the process with the other 3 eggs and egg whites.

USP: An Italian hint to a regular dish that will surely make it both tasty and interesting.

31) Special PB & J Bowl

Serves: 1

Preparation Time: 5 minutes

Ingredients:

½ cup of easy-to-cook oats

- ½ cup of raspberries or strawberries
- 1 tbsp peanut butter
- 1 cup water

Nutrition info:

Protein – 10.8g

Carbohydrates – 42.2g

Fat – 14.4g

Total Kcals – 341.6 Kcals

Method:

Boil the water and add the oats to it. Cook until the oats are softened (should take about 4 minutes).

1. Before the oats are fully cooked, add the remaining ingredients and let it cook for an extra minute. Stir well so the mixture cooks thoroughly and evenly. Serve dish hot.

USP: Makes your regular, often bland breakfast of cereals an interesting one.

32) Meal out of a Fruit Shake

Serves: 1

Preparation Time: 5 minutes

Ingredients:

1/3 cup fresh strawberries

- ¼ cup bananas, chopped
- ½ tbsp almond butter
- 1 scoop of vegetarian protein powder
- ½ cup of almond milk
- Ice as per your choice

Nutrition info:

Protein – 31g

Carbohydrates – 18.9g

Fat – 7.4g

Total Kcals – 266.2

Method:

Add all the ingredients to a smoothie maker or blender and blend well until all they all have been evenly and fully distributed throughout the drink.

1. Serve the drink chilled, topping it off with dry fruits, if preferred.

USP: A fresh drink with frozen or fresh fruits, take a long cold drink in the morning to be off on an energetic start without feeling too full.

33) Vanilla Milkshake

Serves: 1

Preparation Time: 5 minutes

Ingredients:

½ cup frozen bananas, chopped

- ½ tbsp peanut butter
- ½ cup of coconut milk, unsweetened
- 1 heaping tbsp of protein powder
- Water as required
- 1 tsp of vanilla extract

Nutrition info:

Protein – 17.6g

Carbohydrates – 21.8g

Fat – 9g

Total Kcals – 238.6 Kcals

Method:

Add all the ingredients and mix well in a food processor or blender. Blend them well until you get a smooth and lump-free smoothie or drink.

1. Serve cold to chilled, with toppings of dry fruits or a hint of berry sauces.

USP: Another drink that is refreshing and energetic at the same time.

34) Thick Lentil Soup

Serves: 4

Preparation Time: 35 minutes

Ingredients:

1 medium onion, finely chopped

- 2 medium carrots, peeled and finely chopped or coarsely grated
- 1 cup rinsed and dried lentils
- ½ jalapeno, finely chopped
- 1 tbsp fresh ginger, cleaned, peeled and finely chopped
- 2 garlic cloves, finely chopped
- 1 tbsp olive oil
- 1 bay leaf
- 1 can of light coconut milk
- 1 tbsp low sodium soy sauce
- 1/24 tsp cumin
- 3 cups of low sodium vegetable stock (3 cups water, 2 vegetable stock cubes)
- Salt and pepper as per taste
- Fresh coriander sprigs, finely chopped, to be used for garnishing

Nutrition info:

Protein – 36.7g / 9.2g per serving

Carbohydrates – 108g / 27g per serving

Fat – 28g / 7g per serving

Total Kcals – 830.8 Kcals / 207.7 Kcals

Method:

Take a non-stick shallow pan and heat the oil. Add the chopped jalapeno, onion, ginger, carrots and garlic and sauté until the onion turns golden brown. This should take about 3 minutes.

1. Next, add the lentils, bay leaf, cumin, coconut milk and water (or stock) and stir well. When the mixture has been thoroughly mixed, turn the flame low and cover the pan. Let the mixture simmer on low heat for 30 minutes, with an occasional stir or two in between.

2. After the mixture has been well cooked, take the pan off the flames, pour the soup into a bowl and garnish with cilantro, after you have seasoned the soup with soy sauce and added salt and pepper as per your taste.

USP: Although a soup technically, this simple yet delicious dish is as good as a meal's main course dish.

35) Mushroom Chilli, Voodoo Style

Serves: 2

Preparation Time: 35 minutes

Ingredients:

1 tbsp olive oil

- 1 medium courgette, chopped into large pieces or diced
- 1 medium onion finely chopped
- 1 can of pinto beans, rinsed and drained
- 1 medium carrot, also diced
- ½ lb (pound) cremini mushrooms, washed, dried and also diced
- 2 garlic cloves, finely chopped
- 1 bell pepper of any colour, diced
- 2 preserved chipotle peppers, finely cut
- 1 can of whole, peeled tomatoes (preserved)
- ¼ tsp cumin powder or finely ground cumin seeds
- 1 tsp chilli powder
- ½ tsp oregano
- ½ avocado, sliced thinly
- Salt and pepper as per taste

Nutrition info:

Protein – 39.2g / 19.6g per serving

Carbohydrates – 125.8g / 62.9g per serving

Fat – 27.6g / 13.8g per serving

Total Kcals – 908.4 Kcals / 454.2 Kcals per serving

Method:

In a large shallow saucepan or pan, heat the oil over medium-high flame. Once the oil has heated, add the cut onion, mushrooms, zucchini, carrots, garlic and bell pepper and sauté well. The vegetables will turn soft and brown and that is when you will know they are cooked as desired.

1. To this, add the canned tomatoes, broadly crushed with your fingers. Be careful not to finely crush them as we don't want a very even texture made out of the tomatoes; let them be a little pulpy even when crushed. Add the chipotle, chilli powder, cumin, beans and oregano and stir well. Turn the flames to low and cover the dish. Let it simmer so or about 20 minutes. Add

the salt and pepper while the dish simmers.

2. Once fully cooked, pour the dish into bowls, top off with sliced avocados and serve hot.

USP: Filled with exotic flavours and ingredients, this is a must-try dish for people who want the best of health and flavour for lunch or dinner.

36) Creative Salad, Mediterranean Style

Serves : 1

Preparation Time : 5 minutes

Ingredients:

¼ cup cherry tomatoes, in halves

- 4 Kalamata Olives, pitted and halved
- ¼ cup hearts of artichokes
- ¼ cup cooked chickpeas
- 2 cups kale, de-ribbed and cut (Dinosaur Kale preferable)
- 1/8 cup red onion, sliced
- 2 tbsp walnuts, chopped
- 1 tbsp cider vinaigrette
- Sale & pepper

Nutrition info:

Protein – 18.9g

Carbohydrates – 58.5g

Fat – 30.7g

Total Kcals – 585.9 Kcals

Method:

1. Rub the kale to soften the leaves for better texture while chewing and taste.

Mix all ingredients in a large bowl and serve fresh.

USP: Great dish when you want a nutritious snack that's not over-filling.

37) Cashew and Gesundheit

Serves: 4

Preparation Time: 10 minutes

Ingredients:

1/3 cup cashews, chopped, unsalted

- 2 tbsp virgin coconut oil
- 1 lb of chicken breast, de-skinned
- 1 large red bell pepper, chopped and julienned
- 1 tsp minced garlic cloves
- ½ tsp fresh ginger, peeled and finely chopped
- 3 tbsp. spring onion, minced
- 1 cup of brown cooked rice

Nutrition info:

Protein – 167.1g / 41.8g per serving

Carbohydrates – 90.7g / 22.7g per serving

Fat – 86.1g / 21.5g per serving

Total Kcals – 1806.1 Kcals / 451.5 Kcals per serving

Method:

In a large non-stick pan, dry roast chopped cashews until they're lightly toasted, without being burnt. Remove them once so roasted, add coconut oil to the same pan and add chicken strips.

1. Sauté the strips for 2 minutes, add ginger and garlic after 2 minutes and cook for another 30 seconds.
2. Then add all the remaining ingredients, except rice, and cook for about another minute. Serve the dish hot with the cooked rice.

USP: A filling meal with natural flavours of cashew.

38) Amazing Burger

Serves: 4
Preparation Time: 15 minutes
Ingredients:
1 lb lean beef mince
- 1 cup sliced mushrooms
- ½ cup caramelized onions
- 4 gluten-free buns
- 1 tsp freshly cracked pepper
- 1 tsp salt
- 2 cups arugula lettuce
- Mustard and Ketchup as per choice and taste

Nutrition info:
Protein – 117.6g / 29.4g per serving

Carbohydrates – 173.6g / 43.4g per serving

Fat – 60.9g / 15.2g per serving

Total Kcals – 1712.9 Kcals / 428.2 Kcals per serving

Method:
Make 4 patties by mixing the beef, pepper and salt and then frying is just right on a

grill. The insides should be yieldingly soft while the outer side of the patties are firm and cooked. This should take about 3 minutes each side.

1. Sauté sliced mushrooms in olive oil until they release some water. Lightly toast the buns and cut them into halves.
2. On the lower halves, equally distribute arugula, the mushrooms and grilled meat. Cover with other half and serve with mustard and/or ketchup, if required.

USP: A great fulfilling snack while you're on the move.

39) Chicken with Barley and Chilli

Serves: 4

Preparation Time: 4 hours 15 minutes

Ingredients:

2 chicken breasts

- 3 garlic cloves, minced
- 1 cup pearled barley
- ½ onion, minced
- 1 can kidney beans
- 3 tbsp. tomato paste
- 2 cans chopped tomatoes
- 3 cups kale
- 30g grated cheddar cheese, low fat
- Pinch of oregano, salt & pepper

Nutrition info:

Protein – 114.8g / 28.7g per serving

Carbohydrates – 175.1g / 43.8g per serving

Fat – 17.3g / 4.3g per serving

Total Kcals – 1315.3 Kcals / 328.8 per serving

Method:

In a vessel on medium high flames, heat oil and then add chicken breasts with diced tomatoes, onion, garlic, barley, beans, oregano and tomato paste. Let this mixture cook for 3 hours and then add de-ribbed kale leaves.

1. Let it cook for another hour and then serve dish hot.

USP: Tangy flavour with meat and nutrient dense.

40) Chicken Salad with Berries and Citrus

Serves: 4

Preparation Time: 35 minutes

Ingredients:

A pound of de-skinned and boneless chicken breasts

- ½ ounce chicken broth
- ½ cup strawberries, chopped
- 1/3 cup orange juice
- 2 tbsp. olive oil
- 1 tsp sugar
- 1 tbsp lemon juice
- 2 tsp shredded lemon zest
- ¼ tsp salt
- ½ tsp chilli powder
- ¼ tsp pepper (freshly ground)
- 6 cups leafy vegetables, chopped (spinach, kale, watercress, etc.)
- ¼ cup toasted walnuts, chopped

Nutrition info:

Protein – 150.8g / 37.7g per serving

Carbohydrates – 72.8g / 18.2g per serving

Fat – 47.8g / 11.9g per serving

Total Kcals – 1325.2 Kcals / 331.3 Kcals per serving

Method:

Boil chicken broth and add chicken breasts coated with pepper and salt. Let it simmer for 20 minutes, covered and then remove chicken from broth.

1. In a blender, mix strawberries, orange juice, lemon juice and peel, sugar, salt, chilli powder, black pepper and salad oil. Make a fine juice and then add to chicken. Let this mixture simmer or about 5 minutes, uncovered.

2. Once fully cooked, serve sliced chicken with remaining ingredients such as greens and salad greens. Sprinkle walnuts and some dressing if required and serve dish at room temperature.

USP: A unique blend of citric fruits with meat.

The juice section

Method: The following recipes will only list the ingredients required. The procedure to prepare the juices would be the same – blend all ingredients together to make the juice.

41) Cucumber and Tomato

Ingredients:

3 ½ cups tomatoes

- 2 cups cucumber
- 1 celery stalk
- Few stevia drops
- ½ tsp black pepper, ground
- ¼ tsp cayenne pepper
- ½ tsp sea salt

Nutrition info:

Protein – 7.2g

Carbohydrates – 36.4g

Fat – 1.6g

Total Kcals – 188.8 Kcals

42) Carrot and Watercress

Ingredients:

1 cup watercress, chopped
- 2 medium sized carrots
- 2 tomatoes
- ½ cup spinach
- 1 tsp kosher salt
- 1 tsp ground black pepper
- ½ cup cilantro

Nutrition info:

Protein – 4.6g

Carbohydrates – 22.8g

Fat – 0.9g

Total Kcals – 117.7 Kcals

43) Beet and Celery

Ingredients:

5 celery stalks
- 1 bunch cilantro
- 1 small cut beet
- 1 cup spinach, cut

Nutrition info:

Protein – 4.3g

Carbohydrates – 23.2g

Fat – 1.7g

Total Kcals – 125.3 Kcals

44) Spinach with Apples

Ingredients:

2 cups chopped spinach

- ½ cup red lettuce leaves or carrot greens
- 3 medium apples, chopped
- ½ tsp lemon juice
- Cayenne pepper and kosher salt to taste

Nutrition info:

Protein – 3g

Carbohydrates – 60.2g

Fat – 0.9g

Total Kcals – 260.9 Kcals

45) Grapefruit Juice

Ingredients:
1 grapefruit
- 1 yellow pepper
- 1 small, cut beet
- 3 large carrots
- 1 small kiwi
- 7 drops stevia
- ½" peeled ginger

Nutrition info:
Protein – 8.6g

Carbohydrates – 80.7g

Fat – 1.8g

Total Kcals – 373.4 Kcals

46) **Mini Cake Sandwiches**

Serves – 10

Preparation Time - 20 minutes

Ingredients:

½ cup skim milk, divided

- 1 egg white
- ½ cup low fat cream cheese
- 2 tbsp confectioner's sugar
- ½ tsp. Vanilla extract
- ½ cup non-fat Greek yoghurt
- ¾ cup all purpose flour
- ¼ cup unsweetened cocoa powder and a tbsp more for dusting
- ½ cup granulated sugar
- ½ tsp baking soda
- 3 tbsp unsalted butter
- Cooking spray

Nutrition info:

Protein – 53.8g / 5.4g per serving

Carbohydrates – 218.5g / 21.8g per serving

Fat – 66.1g / 6.6g per serving

Total Kcals – 1684.1 Kcals / 168.4 Kcals per serving

Method:

In a large bowl, blend or mix well with an electric mixer the cream cheese and confectioner's sugar until soft and fluffy. To this, add yoghurt and vanilla and mix well.

1. Heat oven at 400 degrees F and line 3 baking sheets with cooking spray. In a separate bowl, mix cocoa powder and baking soda. In a third bowl, mix sugar and butter with egg white until they are well mixed and the mixture turns slightly yellow and thick. Add the flour mixture to the bowl in which you mixed butter and beat well. Add ¼ of the milk and gently mix all ingredients.

2. Do the same with the flour mixture and remaining milk. Pour this mixture into a big, re-saleable bag and tie it up in such a way that it can be used as a piping bag.

3. Make 16 batter lines, about 4" long and about an inch apart on the sprayed and lined baking sheets. Bake the lines until

the centre o the lines rise, are soft and spring back when touched. Place them on the cooling rack.

4. Cut them into smaller sizes, add the cheese mixture on half of them, top them with the other half, dust with cocoa powder and your cake-sandwiches are ready to be served.

USP: This yummy, sweet yet low-calorie snack is great for chocolate lovers who are trying to shed some weight without giving up on their love for chocolate.

47)
Apple Chips

Serves: 4

Preparation time: 1 hour and 40 minutes

Ingredients:

4 crisp red apples, sliced in the shape of chips, each chip being 1/8**th** of an inch thick

- 2 tbsp sugar
- 1/8 tsp cinnamon

Nutrition info:

Protein – 2.2g / 0.5g per serving

Carbohydrates – 177.8g / 44.4g per serving

Fat – 1.4g / 0.3g per serving

Total Kcals – 732.6 Kcals / 183.1 Kcals

Method:

Pre-heat an oven to 225 degrees F. In a bowl, mix the sugar and cinnamon.

1. On lined baking sheets, place the apple chips and sprinkle the sugar mixture. Bake them for an hour. Remove the baking sheets, remove the apple chips

and replace them on the same sheets. Return them peeled and restored to the oven and bake for another 30 minutes.

2. Remove chips and serve hot or preserve for up to 5 days in an airtight bag or container.

USP: Sweet yet healthy snack

48) Beet Soup with Chives and Orange Scent

Serves: 4

Preparation Time: 1 hour and five minutes

Ingredients:

2 ounces of goat cheese

- 2 tbsp fresh chives, chopped
- 2 tbsp balsamic vinegar
- 2 tsp lemon juice
- ¼ tsp salt
- ½ cup orange juice
- ¼ cup minced shallots
- Grated zest of 1 orange
- 2 cans of sliced beets, drained (keep the preserve liquid in a cup)
- 1 crisp red apple, cored, peeled and cut into chunks
- 1 tsp brown sugar

Nutrition info:

Protein – 35.2g / 8.8g per serving

Carbohydrates – 292.6g / 73.1g per serving

Fat – 13.4g / 3.3g per serving
Total Kcals – 1431.8 Kcals / 357.9 Kcals

Method:

In a food processor, add the cut apples, shallots, zest, sugar, salt and beet and make puree. Add the preserve liquid to the puree and mix them all well until an even mixture is formed.

1. Pour mixture in a bowl; add vinegar, lemon juice and orange juice. Cover the bowl and chill in a refrigerator until its cold.
2. Pour chilled soup into 4 bowls, top each off with cut chives and grated cheese to serve.

USP: A tangy, wholesome cold soup with a unique blend of ingredients

49)
Spicy Tacos with Lentil

Serves: 4

Preparation Time: 40 minutes

Ingredients:

½ cup low fat cheddar, shredded

- 1 cup tomatoes, chopped
- 1 cup minced lettuce
- 8 taco shells
- ¼ cup fat-free sour cream
- 2 tsp adobo sauce
- 1 chipotle chilli in adobo sauce (reduce quantity if less spicy preferred)
- 2 ½ cups of vegetable broth
- 1 tbsp olive oil
- 1 cup minced onion
- ½ tsp salt
- 1 minced garlic clove
- 1 cup dried brown lentils, rinsed
- 1 packet taco seasoning, Old El Paso

Nutrition info:

Protein – 131.3g / 32.8g per serving

Carbohydrates – 285.6g / 71.4g per serving

Fat – 74.4g / 18.6g per serving

Total Kcals – 2337.2 Kcals / 584.3 Kcals per serving

Method:

Heat oil in large non-stick pan or skillet. Add salt, onion and garlic. Fry until onion golden brown. Add taco seasoning and lentils to oil. Stir to cook until lentils are dry (takes about a minute). Pour vegetable broth into pan and boil the mixture.

1. Reduce flames and cover the pan. Cook on simmer for 25 minutes until lentils soften. In a separate bowl, mix the chilli, adobo sauce and sour cream.

2. Uncover pan, pour the lentil mixture equally into taco shells. Top it with the cream mixture, shredded lettuce, cheese and tomato.

USP: Healthy option for junk food lovers

Recipe 50 – Zingy Berries' Smoothie

Serves: 1

Preparation Time: 10 minutes

Ingredients:

¼ cup oats

- ¼ cup 1% low fat milk
- ½ tsp fresh ginger, grated
- 1 cup blackberries, fresh
- ¼ cup strawberries, sliced
- 1 tsp honey
- ½ cup ice

Nutrition info:

Protein – 8.4g

Carbohydrates – 49.8g

Fat – 3.7g

Total Kcals – 266.1 Kcals

Method:

Take all ingredients, add to blender and mix well.

1. Serve with ice

Part 2

Introduction

I want to thank you and congratulate you for purchasing the book, "Low Carb Diet: The Best Guide To Low Carb - Lose Fat And Get A Fast Metabolism In 7 Days With This Weight Loss Blood Sugar Solution Diet!".

This book contains proven steps and strategies on how to get the body of your dreams!

Don't let another week pass you by living life out of shape! The extra weight around your waistline or hips is more than just a problem of how you look in the mirror. Especially if it is not burned off in the near future, it can cause a host of other problems relating to your health and longevity. You owe it to yourself and the ones close to you to get in the best shape of your life.

Imagine how nice it would feel to look in the mirror and be happy with what you see on the outside and be comforted knowing that you are much healthier on the inside.

If you are serious about finally losing weight and keeping it off, then you have come to the right place. "Low Carb Diet: Low Carb Diet Solution - In as Little as 7 Days You Can Lose Weight Fast Using This Low Carb Diet Plan!" is the solution you have been looking for that allows you to literally create the body of your dreams, and what's even better is you will start seeing results within the first 7 days. Anyone who truly wants to lose weight can use these principles and be on their way in a matter of days! Don't waste another week, begin living life to the fullest today!

This book does not offer a drastic solution. But it will show you how to customize your low carb meals for seven days so you can start experiencing your desired weight loss results.

Thanks again for purchasing this book, I hope you enjoy it!

Chapter 1 – What Is A Low Carb Diet?

I am so excited for you! If you are reading this far, it means that you truly are looking for change in your life! You are tired of not living to your full potential, and ready to start living the way you were intended to. That's great, and what better way to start than by creating the best body of your life!

Keep that enthusiasm high because that is exactly what will carry you through to reaching your goals. The truth is the most important factor in your goals being obtained is you. You are the one that must "decide". You must simply make a choice that no matter what, you will reach your goal. If you simply do this, than I am confident you will succeed.

So let's get started! But Before we jump straight into what you should eat and the details of the diet, we need to make sure you are caught up to speed on the basics of a low carb diet.

If you've been dieting or have at least tried to do something about your weight, then you might have heard or read about low carb diets. Some of the popular fad-diets that can be classified as low carb diets include Sugar Busters Diet, the well-known South Beach Diet, the ever popular Zone Diet, Atkins, and pretty much every other diet you may have heard of.

As you should know by now, the term "low carb diet" has actually been applied to many different diets. It's a really broad classification of different diets that limit carbohydrate intake. Some people call them low glycemic diets while others refer to them as reduced carbohydrate diets.

The common denominator for these diets that belong to the "low carb" class is that they require, just as the name suggests, a diet that excludes foods that are heavy in carbohydrates. These are foods that are referred to as glycemic. There are lists of foods and their glycemic index to guide people going on any low carb diet.

So How Low Carb is Low Carb, Really?

You may consult your doctor about how low carb your diet should be; this is the smartest thing you should do before engaging in any diet. The dietary guidelines in the United States state that around 50 to 65 percent of a person's calorie intake for any given day should come from carbs.

Generally speaking, you should simply have less than 50% to 65% calories coming from carbohydrate sources of any variant in your daily diet. There are low carb diets that recommend only 20% or less of your daily caloric intake. If you want to live off a low carb diet for weight loss, keeping your carbohydrate intake to less than 20% of your daily caloric requirement is advised. Of course, you should make sure that you substitute this with another calorie source, mostly vegetables. With this kind of drastic drop in carbohydrate consumption, not all people are able to handle the dietary changes.

Your body will react. You can feel uneasy because of cravings for the carbs that you are used to having. That is why you will have to slowly adjust your carb intake up to the point when your body can take the loss of carbs. You may think that's a bit of a hit and miss approach, but the fact remains that everyone has a different tolerance for carb loss.

Chapter 2 – Different Approaches To

Achieve Ideal Results

Notice that different low carb diets will use different approaches to achieve the desired effects. One approach is to simply just reduce a person's carb intake immediately. The idea behind this approach is pretty basic: the fewer carbs you take in the fewer calories you gain, period.

If you count calories and check out the numbers, then this approach may sound very plausible. These kinds of diets usually advise against adding sugars or using refined carb sources.

The methodology is simple. All you have to do is to get rid of the side orders, extra helpings, and meal add-ons in your diet that tend to bloat your calorie intake. Another way to apply this approach is to

116

simply get rid of the white foods you usually eat like white flour, white refined sugar, rice and any other white grains, and potatoes (white or yellow ones included).

The next approach is to determine just how much carbs each dieter needs to take off his meals in order to lose weight. This method is less drastic and a lot safer for people. It follows the idea that each person has a different carb tolerance. Older people have a harder time digesting carbs. The objective in this approach is to define the optimal carb level for each individual. This is basically one of the ideas behind the South Beach Diet and similar diets.

The last approach is to teach your body to use the calories from stores in your body fat. Your body is naturally attuned to using fat in order to gain energy. It will take time for your body to stop making use of glucose and concentrate on the use of stored fat in the body. This process is called ketosis.

Diets that make use of this bodily process are called ketonic diets. Note that some ketonic diets are applied by some medical experts to treat chronic diseases such as epilepsy. However, when this approach is applied to weight loss, it is referred to by such experts as James Volek and Stephen Phinneyas nutritional ketosis. One of the phases of the Atkins diet is actually ketogenic in nature. This approach is not suited for everyone, but there are people who have become quite successful at losing weight using ketonic diets.

During the initial stages of ketosis the brain will refrain from burning ketones. Doing so, the body will stop making use of stored glycogen but will instead concentrate on making use of stored body fat. In this mode, your body will make use of stored carbs only when it is absolutely necessary. This also helps prevent your body from eating up the stored proteins found in your muscles.

Chapter 3 – The Case Of The Atkins Diet:

To Be Strict Or Not

In this Chapter, we'll look into one of the low carb diets that have become popular in recent years, the Atkins Diet. We'll look into its pros and cons and we'll allow you to decide if it is the right one for you.

The Atkins Diet has four stages or phases: Induction, Ongoing Weight Loss, Pre-Maintenance, and Maintenance. There is no set pattern on which phase one should start with. However, it is highly encouraged that people begin with the Induction Phase since it will prepare the body for the drop in carbohydrates. This is also the phase where ketosis occurs since your body will be induced or forced into burning fat stores rather than glycogen stores.

Looking Into the Induction Phase

This Phase will help you figure out your carb tolerance level. Once you know how many carbs you can basically live with, the diet will then adjust to how your body behaves. You will have to determine how much carbs you can bear losing. Once that level is determined, dieters will then monitor carb intake and maintain the level where they are able to successfully lose weight. The Induction lasts for a period of two weeks but staying on it longer is also encouraged.

Foods Allowed

Dieters going through the Atkins diet should avoid refined sources of carbs. You can eat any carb source that is nutrient dense. Just like any low carb diet out there, the emphasis in food choice has to do with smartly choosing your sources of carbohydrates.

Dieters are supposed to get most of their carbs from vegetables. Dieters are allowed

12 to 15 grams of vegetables each day. They are also allowed to consume protein as well as fats. Most types of cheeses are allowed, but not fresh cheeses such as farmer's cheese or cottage cheese. Dieters are allowed only three to four ounces of cheese each day.

Protein sources such as eggs, meat, and seafood are okay. You are also allowed to eat plenty of omega 3 fatty acid sources (e.g. cold water fish etc.). Olive oil, grape seed oil, peanut oil, and canola oil are also allowed. Surprisingly, regular full fat mayonnaise is allowed as well as butter.

When it comes to beverages, water is number one (this is basically the case for any low carb diet). Any beverage that has sugar in it is not allowed. However, diet sodas that are sweetened using Splenda (sucralose) are allowed. Splenda and Sweet n Low (saccharine) are your basic sweeteners while on this diet. Low carb snacks are allowed but you should check the label for sugar content.

The Pros and Cons of the Induction Phase

The induction phase of the Atkins Diet has received a lot of negative criticism even from proponents of low carb dieting. They cite the fact that it is too restrictive. If you look at the earlier books on the Atkins Diet, they stress this phase as an extremely important part of the Diet. Nowadays, however, Atkins Diet authors tend to veer away from such assertions.

The good side of this phase is that it jump starts you into the very heart of low carb dieting. You'll be giving up a lot of carbs in the onset. If you are used to eating a lot of carbs, then this phase will allow you to make a 180 degree turn towards the other direction. It sort of drastically changes your eating habits right smack into what healthy eating should be.

On the bad side, this diet presents a radical dietary change that might not be tolerable for some people. However, experts say that you can actually start on a carb level that is higher than what the Induction Phase recommends. You can simply work on a gradual decrease of carbohydrates as you progress in the diet.

More Pros and Cons of Low Carb Diets

Aside from possibly getting a carb crashas mentioned above, there are some other negatives about the Atkins Diet that you should know about. As it has come under scrutiny, you might have heard about a number of both positive and negative things about it, including myths and misconceptions.

One of the popular comments about the Atkins Diet is that counting carbs is a meticulous process which requires a lot of planning. Once you have gotten the hang of low carb meal planning, however, you will not have to do a lot of counting anymore.

Boredom is another common negative among all low carb diets. With very few food choices, some people eventually get bored with the diet. The answer to this is a lot of creativity in meal options and low carb recipes.

Moving on to the positive side of this diet, people who love their steak and butter will be happy to note that these foods that are often forbidden in other diets are back on the menu. While this diet is restrictive when it comes to carbs and sugars, it is actually quite lenient on the other tasty treats that you normally crave for. That being said, it should be noted that dieters are still supposed to consume a variety of fats, which include healthy fats such as the ones from olive oil etc.

The Atkins Diet as well as other low carb diets is pretty easy to learn. Once you learn how to count carbs and identify the foods you can eat, you don't have to think much about everything else. Another good thing about low carb diets in general is that you are encouraged to find your own carbohydrate sensitivity. You get to determine just how much carbs you need to remove from your diet and how much you can tolerate.

Chapter 4 – What Does A Low Carb Diet Look Like?

So, what does a low carb diet meal look like? The following are breakfast options, lunch options, dinner options, and snack options that you will find in many low carb diet plans. If you want to try living a slightly low carb diet than the one you're in right now, I suggest that you plan your meals for 7 days and choose from the following options.

Breakfast Options

The following are breakfast options that you can mix and match. You will still be able to have bread, eggs, and cereals for breakfast. The big difference is that they won't be that heavy in their carb content.

Breads: bread, muffins, or biscuits made from low carb ingredients such as almond meal or flax meal. If you miss pancakes, you can find low carb pancake mixes too.

Low Carb Cereals: choose high fiber cereals like Fiber One. Check the label and make sure that cereals you choose are truly low carb.

Eggs: The easiest way to cook eggs is to boil them. Note that one hardboiled egg contains 0.5 grams of net carbs. But that is not always a tasty treat. To add flavor to eggs, turn them into an omelet with some left over veggies tossed into the mix.

Low Carb Fruit Breakfast: Fruits are a great low carb breakfast option. Examples of which include blackberries, cranberries, and lemons. The following fruits have medium sugar content: peaches, grapefruit, strawberries, apricots, papaya, guavas, cantaloupes, apples, casaba melons, honeydew melons, water melons, blueberries, and nectarines.

Now there are fruits that have higher sugar content, so be careful with these: pineapple, pears, plums, kiwifruit, and oranges. The following fruits should rarely be eaten. If you do, you should reduce your carb intake from other sources. The fruits with high sugar content are as follows: bananas, tangerines, mangoes, cherries, figs, and grapes.

Spoonable Breakfasts: Let's face it. There are mornings when you'll be in a hurry and won't have time to prepare a low carb meal. You can go pick some of the fruit mentioned above and you can add some of the following: ricotta cheese, yogurt, and cottage cheese. That's a pretty tasty quick breakfast you can spoon to your heart's content.

Lunch Ideas

Lunch is one of the important meals of the day. It's your mid-way break in your eight hour work day or school day. Lunches are often done in a hurry. Those who do not have time to prepare their lunch would be constrained to go for fast food which normally consists of a burger, a big-sized soda, and some fries on the side. This lunch is eaten just as fast as it is ordered. It does not take a dietitian to say that this is not healthy at all.

You basically have to try to deviate from the usual lunch ideas and stick to healthier food choices that are low in carbs. You'll get the energy that you need to complete your day without loading up on the fats that make you gain weight. The options below will give you a lot to choose from when planning your week's lunches. They are relatively easy to prepare and they taste just as good as any good old lunch you ever had.

Salad not Sandwich

Many people grew up with the idea of having sandwiches for lunch. A couple of slices of white bread with veggies and meat in between would have been the perfect lunch if you're not overweight. If you're trying to lose weight, you better skip the white bread and stick to the stuff sandwiched in the middle.

Go with veggies, cheese, and meat. When you think about it, this suggestion sounds more like a salad. Salads are the best way to go when you're making lunch on the go even if you're on a low carb diet.

Salad Options: The most common salad option is the good old chef's salad: one serving of iceberg lettuce (the size of a tennis ball) chopped, one hardboiled egg, chopped cold cuts, and a sprinkle of cheese. That already looks great and it's a great weight loss option too. However, it won't be too appetizing if you have that for lunch every day for seven days.

The good news is that there are a lot of salad options for lunch when you're on a low carb diet. When choosing salad greens, it is better to go for the darker greens. They are definitely more nutritious. At least you know which kind of bagged greens you're supposed to get from the grocery store.

A bunch of leaves with spices and a few other vegetables don't make a mean salad. What really makes a salad a true blue salad is the dressing. However, not every dressing will work wonders for your low carb diet. The following salad dressings will work best for your low carb diet plan:

Caesar Salad Dressing: 0.5 gram net carbs

Oil and Vinegar: 1 gram net carbs

Ranch: 1.4 grams net carbs

Blue Cheese: 2.3 grams net carbs

Lime Juice: 2.8 grams net carbs

Lemon Juice: 2.8 grams net carbs

Italian Dressing: 3 grams net carbs

NOTE: All servings on this list are 2 tablespoons. Don't add sugar to dressing.

With the many salad greens as well as dressing options available you can make the following salads: Thai chicken salad, Greek salad, tuna salad, chopped salad with chicken, blanched greens with salmon, and low carb taco salad among many others.

Slightly Heavier Lunch Options: There are folks who want a slightly heavier lunch, which is understandable if you're going on a low carb diet for the very first time. There are lunch options that are great for dieters who want to avoid a lot of carbs.

The following are some of your best lunch options for heavier low carb meals:

Baked salmon (200 grams), snow peas, spring greens, and a drizzle of lemon juice.

Diced seasonal veggies (1 cup), miso soup (225 ml).

Grilled chicken (180 grams) with a light drizzle of fresh squeezed lemon juice, whole grain rice (1 cup).

One serving of miso soup (300 ml), grilled tofu and bokchoy (100 grams).

Baked chicken (180 grams without skin) with vinaigrette flavoring (15 ml).

Canned tuna (95 grams), diced onions, lettuce (1 cup), and lemon zest.

Sourdough (1 piece), scrambled eggs (2 pieces), half a cup diced tomatoes.

Cooked quinoa (1 cup), steamed broccoli (one cup), walnuts (10 grams).

Pan fried steak (5 ounces), mushroom (1 cup) plus herbs, steamed green beans (1 cup).

Burgers (minus the buns); you can go to your favorite burger place, order bun-less burgers or just remove the burgers yourself. Don't get any extra orders on the side like French fries or onion rings and you shouldn't get any sweetened drink – just water will do.

Dinner Options

Dinners can be tempting especially if you have your carb reduced dishes served alongside what the rest of the family is eating. Sometimes, losing weight is a lonely enterprise. You need the help and support of the entire family especially come dinner time when all of you are gathered around the dinner table. If you're lucky enough to get the family on the same ground, you can all have the same low carb meal during dinner.

The following are tasty dinner options that are definitely low carb. They are delectable enough so that the rest of the family can enjoy the same dishes with you. You can create your meal plans for an entire week and pick from any of the dishes mentioned here.

Baked Meatballs

You only need half a pound each of ground pork, ground round, and ground lamb. You'll also need one egg, chopped spinach (5 ounces), 1 teaspoon garlic (minced), 1 teaspoon salt, 1 teaspoon dried basil, half a teaspoon of crushed pepper, and half a cup of bread crumbs.

You just have to mix everything up, except for the bread crumbs of course. Place the mixture in the fridge and leave it there for 24 hours. Take it out the next evening, preheat your oven to 400 degrees Fahrenheit. Turn the mixture into 1.5 ounce balls, roll them over the bread crumbs, place them on a sheet, and bake them for 20 minutes. You can place the balls in individual muffin cups if you like.

One serving will have about four meatballs. It only yields 10 grams of carbs! This meal also provides you with 432 calories. Now, even your kids won't complain about this low carb menu item.

Spaghetti Squash

There's always room for spaghetti in low carb menus. You'll be cooking spaghetti the same old way except that instead of using the usual pasta you're going to use spaghetti squash, which has lower carb content. Regular pasta will give you 42 grams of carbs per serving while spaghetti squash will only yield 10 grams of carbs per serving. You will also have a full tummy with just 42 calories in your spaghetti squash low carb dinner.

Cauliflower Chowder

This is not a pure cauliflower recipe, so you don't have to worry about stuffing yourself with a single veggie. You'll need five slices of bacon (chopped), onion powder (1 teaspoon), 1 stalk of celery (chopped), water (2 tablespoons), flour (2 tablespoons), salt and pepper, shredded cauliflower (4 cups), shredded cheddar cheese (12 ounces), 2 chopped green onions, and 2 cups of chicken broth.

Mix together one quarter chicken broth plus flour and set it aside. Sauté bacon, and place on paper towels when crispy to remove excess fat. Sauté onions, garlic, and celery; season with salt and pepper.

After that, you can add the cauliflower, chicken broth, water, and milk, and bring it to a boil. Add in the flour and chicken broth mixture and simmer for 3 minutes or until the chowder has thickened. You may then add the bacon and cheddar cheese. You can top the chowder with either drops of hot sauce or chopped green onions.

This recipe makes a total of eight servings. It only provides seven grams of carbs and it makes a very satisfying dinner.

Other Dinner Ideas: There are a lot of low carb dinner ideas to come and you definitely won't miss the carbs once you're full these really tasty and satisfying foods. Here are some more dinner ideas for low carb diets:

- Baked salmon (200 grams)
- Canned tuna (95 grams)
- Grilled chicken (180 grams)
- Grilled tofu (100 grams)
- Grilled trout (200 grams)
- Mixed beans salad

Veggie Food Options

When you're going for a 7 day low carb menu plan, you should replace the bulk of the carbs you usually eat with veggies. It is recommended that you consume around

12 to 15 grams of net carbs coming from vegetables. A serving would be about the size of a tennis ball. Here are some quick bits of info that you can use when preparing veggies for your meals:

- Alfalfa sprouts: serving size 16 grams; 0.2 g net carbs
- Asparagus: serving size 6 spears; 2.4 g net carbs
- Artichoke hearts: serving size 1 can; 1 g net carbs
- Broccoli: serving size 80 grams; 1.7 g net carbs
- Celery: serving size 1 stalk; 0.4 g net carbs
- Chives: serving size 1 tablespoon; 0.1 g net carbs
- Cauliflower: serving size 60 grams; 1.4 net carbs
- Bok Choy: serving size 70 grams; 0.4 g net carbs
- Iceberg lettuce: serving size 70 grams; 0.2 g net carbs

- Romaine lettuce: serving size 45 grams; 0.4 g net carbs
- Mushrooms: serving size 35 grams; 1.2 g net carbs
- Kale: serving size 65 grams; 2.4 g net carbs
- Leeks: serving size 50 grams; 3.4 g net carbs
- Green string beans: serving size 100 grams; 4.1 g net carbs
- Green olives: serving size 5 pieces; 0.1 g net carbs
- Black olives: serving size 5 pieces; 0.7 g net carbs
- Sauerkraut: serving size 70 grams; 1.2 g net carbs
- Onion: serving size 20 grams; 4.3 g net carbs
- Spaghetti squash: serving size 40 grams when boiled; 2.0 g net carbs
- Okra: serving size 80 grams; 2.4 g net carbs
- Spinach: serving size 90 grams; 2.2 g net carbs

- Snow peas: serving size 60 grams; 3.4 g net carbs
- Tomatoes: serving size 60 grams; 4.3 g net carbs

Snack Options

In case you find yourself hungry at any point in your low carb dieting, you may want to gobble up some snacks to curb the craving without putting on more carbs. You may include any of the following in your meal plans:

- One apple + 10 cashews
- 1 banana + 10 cashews
- One banana + 5 Brazil nuts
- Liver cleanse juice (ginger root, beetroot, ½ regular size carrot, and celery)
- 10 cashews
- 30grams of hummus + 1 piece of unrefined whole wheat pita bread

- 30grams of mixed dried fruit (watch the sugar content)
- 1 whole wheat pita with ¼ avocado
- One regular sized banana
- 1 orange + 5 Brazil nuts (just have to love Brazil)
- 30grams hummus + carrot sticks
- 1 chopped carrot + 4 olives
- Banana Strawberry Shake (cheat treat – use only once a week!)

Chapter 5 – How To Make Your 7 Day Low Carb Meal Plan

This is the point where you will make sense of it all. In the previous chapter you have been given a list of food items, meals, and recipes that you can make in order to get you started on a low carb diet.

The next step is to make a meal plan for days one to seven. Choose a breakfast option for each of the seven days. Choose a lunch option for each day. And choose a lunch option for each day.

The 6 Hour Secret

Now, the idea is to not go hungry within a six hour period. You're used to eating lots of carbs during the day and a good strategy to help you overcome any hunger pangs and cravings is to have low carb snacks ready for consumption within any six hour period.

When it comes to snacks, you can just wing it or make a schedule just like what you did for breakfast, lunch, and dinner. Have a good low carb drink ready in a drink bottle so you don't get tempted to grab a can of soda or any sugary drink. If you must sweeten your drink, make sure that you use Splenda (sucralose) or Sweet n Low (saccharine).

Sample Single Day Meal Plan

Breakfast: Sourdough toast (1 slice only) + 50 grams of ricotta; drizzle with 2 tablespoons honey

Snack: Carrot sticks and hummus

Lunch: Canned tuna (95 grams) + diced lemons and lettuce

Snack: 30 grams mixed dried fruit + cashews (10 pieces)

Dinner: Grilled chicken (180 grams) with steamed broccoli.

Drinks during the day: tea (sweetened with Splenda if desired), water (eight glasses)

Conclusion

Thank you again for purchasing this book on the best way to implement a Low Carb Diet in your eating program!

I hope this book was able to help you to gain insights about the principles of a low carb diet and the strategies that you can use to achieve the body that you have been dreaming of.

The next step is to get started!

The tips in this book won't give you drastic results. What you have been given are flexible and doable strategies to get you started on a low carb diet. Putting these strategies to practice is up to you. How dedicated you are with your diet strategies will determine your success. The low carb diet works, but only if you stick to what it requires.

Once you are comfortable with the lenient and easy to follow low carb strategy described in this book, you can move on to more restrictive diets if you wish to achieve faster results. The important thing is to condition your body to a low carb diet or at least a semi-restricted carb diet. Once you have taken that first step, you can move on to further weight loss using more stringent low carb diet solutions.

About The Author

Marco Barrett loves low carb cooking The author has written several recipe books on the topic. He has served as an instructor promoting various cusine arts in indie shows and fairs. He is currently living with his spouse in Texas.

Lightning Source UK Ltd.
Milton Keynes UK
UKHW020638180722
406010UK00010B/1419

9 781989 749258